David Vau

Recipes to Kill Cancer

A Real Food Guide to Take Your Life Back

Disclaimer

This book is intended for informational and educational purposes only. It is not a substitute for professional medical advice, diagnosis, or treatment. Always seek the advice of your physician or other qualified health provider with any questions you may have regarding a medical condition or before starting any new medical routine, supplement, or lifestyle change. Never disregard professional medical advice or delay seeking it because of something you have read in this book. The author is not a doctor, and the strategies in this book are shared as general guidance. Individual results may vary.

Table Of Contents

Disclaimer 2

A Message From David 5

Chapter 1 7

What Causes Cancer (And How We Got Here) 7

Chapter 2 9

The Stress–Cancer Connection 9

Chapter 3 11

Finding Your Root Cause 11

Chapter 4 13

Making the Choice to Change 13

Chapter 5 15

Fasting — A Secret Weapon 15

Chapter 6 17

Welcome to Your New Life (And New Food) 17

Chapter 7 19

Foods to Pause (Even If They're Healthy) 19

Chapter 8 21

Cancer's Favorite Foods 21

Recipes to Kill Cancer A Real Food Guide to Take Your Life Back

Chapter 9 23

Why Food Can Kill Cancer 23

Chapter 10 26

The Anti-Cancer Vegetable List 26

Chapter 11 28

The Anti-Cancer Fruit List 28

Chapter 12 30

Recipes to Kill Cancer 30

A Message From David

Welcome, If you're holding this book, chances are you — or someone you love — is facing one of life's toughest battles. I know that battle personally. When I was diagnosed with cancer, it shook the ground beneath my feet. Suddenly, life became very real, very fast. I wasn't just fighting for myself — I was fighting for my wife, my children, my grandchildren, and for the life I still had left to live. In those early days, I realized quickly: cancer was not just a physical disease. It was a wake-up call. A wake-up call about what I ate. A wake-up call about how I lived. A wake-up call about the things I thought were healthy — but weren't. I didn't just want treatment. I wanted to rebuild from the inside out. That's where this book was born. Food became one of my greatest weapons — and my greatest healers. I dedicated myself to learning everything I could about what causes cancer, what feeds it, and what starves it. I took everything I learned, tested it through my own journey, and now I'm sharing it here, with you. This is not a book full of trendy diets or magic bullet promises. This is real food, real knowledge, real strength. Inside these pages, you'll find: The root causes behind cancer's rise, How stress, environment, and food choices collide A blueprint for how to take your power back. Recipes made from ingredients that fight, not fuel, disease. Simple tools you can start using today — without feeling overwhelmed.

Whether you are in treatment, recovery, or simply seeking a better path for your health, my hope is that this book gives you something I wish I had on Day One: Clarity. Strength. And hope. You are not powerless. You are not alone. You have more control over your healing

Recipes to Kill Cancer A Real Food Guide to Take Your Life Back

than you've been told. And it can start today — with the next meal you make. —

David Vaughan

Chapter 1

What Causes Cancer (And How We Got Here)

When you hear the word "cancer," it's natural to think it just happens out of nowhere. But the truth is, cancer is rarely random. It's the result of years — sometimes decades of silent damage, hidden stress, and choices we didn't even realize were hurting us. Our modern world looks very different from the one our grandparents grew up in.

Today, we're surrounded by: Processed foods and chemical additives Chronic emotional stress Toxins in the air, water, and products we use every day, Exhaustion and pushing our bodies beyond their limits, Our bodies are incredible. They are built to heal. But even the strongest body can only take so much. I know this now — because for most of my life, I thought strength was enough. I was a professional boxer when I was younger. I trained hard, fought hard, and conditioned myself to handle pain and discomfort. That toughness never really left me. Even a couple of years ago, long after my boxing days had officially ended, I went back into the ring to do some sparring — just to see if I still had it. Physically, I thought I was fine. I was used to pushing through pain. I thought discomfort was normal. But inside, my body was already vulnerable. Decades of heavy bricklaying — a tough, physical job — had worn me down more than I realized. Long hours under the sun, the constant physical strain, the stress that builds up without you even noticing — it all leaves a mark. And somewhere along the way, a seed was planted. Cancer doesn't happen overnight.

It starts small — when the body is weakened, when the internal environment is just right for it to take root. Looking back, I can see now how easy it is to fall into the traps of modern life: Working too hard and resting too little Ignoring the signs our body gives us, Eating foods that damage instead of heal, Carrying stress like a silent weight on our backs, No one ever teaches you how food, stress, and lifestyle collide to create disease.

It's only when something serious happens — like a cancer diagnosis — that we start to connect the dots. But there's power in understanding how we got here. Because if we can see the path we were walking, we can also choose a new one. A path where we: Lighten the toxic load, Strengthen the body's natural defenses, Starve disease instead of feeding it, Create an environment where healing is possible again. This chapter — and this book — isn't about blame or regret.

It's about taking our power back. Not to create fear, but to create hope. Because when you know better, you can do better. And when you do better, you give yourself the best possible chance to heal.

Chapter 2

The Stress–Cancer Connection

If you asked most people what causes cancer, the first answers you'd hear are usually things like smoking, bad diet, or genetics. But there's another powerful, invisible driver that often gets overlooked: Stress. Stress isn't just a feeling — it's a full-body reaction. When you live with ongoing stress, your body releases a constant flood of hormones like cortisol and adrenaline. In the short term, that's fine — it's part of survival. But over the long term, this constant "fight or flight" mode starts breaking your body down: It weakens your immune system It raises inflammation It slows healing It damages your gut lining, where most of your immunity lives In short, chronic stress creates the perfect environment for disease to take hold. Looking back now, I can see how stress was silently running in the background of my own life. As a bricklayer, the work was physically tough — but the mental pressure was just as heavy. Meeting deadlines, keeping jobs flowing, making sure the family was looked after — it all adds up over the years. And like most people, I carried it quietly. I also had a short fuse at times. If something went wrong or frustration built up, I could lose my temper quickly. Every time it happened, I regretted it deeply. I always felt sorry afterward — especially to whoever it was directed at. But in those moments of anger, my body wasn't just reacting emotionally — it was taking a physical hit too.

That sudden rush of adrenaline, that spike in blood pressure, the emotional crash afterward — it was another form of silent stress, weakening my body little by little over the years. You don't realize how much pressure you're carrying until something finally cracks. Then there's emotional stress — the kind that comes from life itself.

Loss, grief, fear, overwork, financial pressure — all of these things don't just sit in your mind. They leave marks on your body too. I was used to pushing through pain. That's what boxing taught me. I thought being tough was about ignoring discomfort.

But the truth is, real strength is recognizing when something is wrong — and doing something about it before it's too late. Stress alone may not cause cancer by itself.

But it weakens the body's natural defenses — making it easier for cancer to take root, grow, and thrive. Learning to manage stress is not a luxury.

It's part of survival. In my own healing journey, managing stress has been just as important as changing what I eat. Slowing down Resting properly Connecting with family Walking outside Doing things that bring peace instead of pressure These aren't just nice ideas. They are part of the work of healing. If you're facing cancer — or trying to prevent it — don't underestimate stress. Finding ways to lighten the load you carry, might just be one of the most powerful medicines you have.

Chapter 3

Finding Your Root Cause

When I was first diagnosed with cancer, I remember asking myself the same question over and over: "How did this happen to me?" I had always thought I was tough. I was used to pain. I was used to discomfort. I worked hard all my life. I provided for my family. I kept moving forward — even when things were hard. But somewhere along the line, something broke down inside my body. And it wasn't just one thing. Cancer doesn't happen because of a single bad meal, a single bad week, or even a single bad year. It builds quietly — over time — from many small factors stacking up on top of each other. That's why, if you truly want to heal, you have to be willing to do something most people never do: You have to find your root cause. Not just the obvious things. Not just the easy answers. You have to dig deep and be brutally honest with yourself: What has my body been exposed to over the years? What kind of food have I fed it most of my life? What levels of stress have I carried — even when I thought I was coping fine? Where have I ignored warning signs because I thought "it's just part of life"? How much real rest, real nutrition, real healing have I given myself over the years? For me, the answers started to become clear the more I sat with them. I could see the years of heavy, physical labour bricklaying. I could see the decades of pushing my body to its limits without proper rest and recovery. I could see the old wounds of stress, pressure, and emotional turmoil that I carried quietly under the surface.

I could see how a diet I thought was "good enough" was actually slowly damaging me from the inside out. It wasn't one thing. It was everything. That's the real truth most people don't want to hear — but it's also the most powerful truth you can accept.

Because once you know what created the problem, you can start to un-create it.

Finding your root cause isn't about blaming yourself. It's about freeing yourself.

It's about facing the reality of where things went wrong — so you can now do everything right. Healing isn't about covering symptoms.

It's about going to the root — digging it out — and giving yourself the chance to rebuild from solid ground. That's what I decided to do. And it started the moment I stopped asking "why me?" And started asking: "What can I change today?"

Chapter 4

Making the Choice to Change

One of the hardest truths about healing is that it's not just about medicine. It's about change. And change is hard. When you first hear the word "cancer," your mind immediately looks outward: "What treatment do I need?" "What doctor can fix this?" "What's the best hospital?" But at some point, if you want real healing, you have to stop looking outward — and start looking inward. You have to ask yourself the question that changes everything: "Am I willing to change my life to save my life?" That's not an easy question to answer. Because changing your life means letting go of old habits. It means challenging what you thought was normal. It means walking a road that most people around you might not understand. I remember having to face this choice head-on. On the outside, people might have seen a strong man — a fighter, a hard worker, someone who could handle anything. But on the inside, I knew that if I kept doing what I had always done, I was going to lose this fight. Cancer was not going to be beaten by doing the same things that helped it grow. I had to change. Completely. I had to change how I saw food. I had to change how I treated my body. I had to change how I handled stress. I had to change my daily routines, my environment, even my thinking. And the hardest part? I had to let go of the belief that I could just "push through it" like I always had before. Healing wasn't about being tougher this time. It was about being wiser. There's a reason why so many people struggle to heal. Change is uncomfortable.

It forces you to slow down, to face the parts of your life you'd rather ignore. It forces you to become someone new — not just survive as who you were. But here's the truth I want you to hold onto: Every small change is a victory. Every better choice you make — every clean meal, every deep breath instead of anger, every act of self-care it all adds up. Healing isn't a one-time event.

Healing is the result of thousands of tiny, courageous choices. You don't have to be perfect. You just have to be willing. Because once you truly make the decision to change, you stop being a victim. You become a fighter again — but this time, a fighter on a much deeper level. This is your life. And it's worth fighting for.

Chapter 5

Fasting — A Secret Weapon

When people think about fighting cancer, the first things that come to mind are usually things like surgery, chemotherapy, and radiation. Very few think about not eating as a weapon. But fasting — done properly — is one of the most powerful tools you have to help your body heal itself. I didn't always know this. Like most people, I grew up believing that eating regularly, keeping your strength up with food, and following the old "three meals a day" rule was just common sense. But cancer doesn't follow common sense. It thrives on certain things — sugar, insulin spikes, constant feeding — and our modern eating habits feed that system perfectly. When I began learning about fasting, everything changed. I discovered that when you stop feeding your body for a time, something incredible happens: Your healthy cells go into a protective, repair mode, Your body burns through damaged cells (including pre-cancerous and cancerous ones) in a process called autophagy, Inflammation drops Insulin levels stabilize, The body can focus its full energy on healing, instead of constantly digesting. In simple terms, fasting starves the disease — while strengthening you. But it's not about starving yourself to weakness. It's about using fasting as a tool, carefully, alongside proper nutrition, hydration, and recovery. After my diagnosis, I made fasting part of my core strategy.

I committed to a 100-hour fast: Starting the day before chemotherapy began, fasting all the way through the chemotherapy treatment, Only breaking the fast after the full chemo cycle finished, The results? I had no symptoms. While many people experience severe nausea, fatigue, pain, and weakness after chemo, also Oxaliplatin is notorious for side effects like cold-triggered nerve tingling, numb fingers and toes, throat tightness with cold drinks, nausea, fatigue, and low blood counts. Many patients also develop longer-term nerve damage after multiple cycles. Remarkably, I experienced almost none of these.

My fasting, clean nutrition, and supportive therapies seemed to protect me, allowing me to sail through treatment without the usual struggles. I experienced none of it. I stayed hydrated with clean water, sea salt, lemon water, and a few cups of green tea with turmeric and black pepper — but I gave my body the space it needed to fight.

Fasting wasn't easy at first. Like most people, I was conditioned to think hunger meant something was wrong. But once I understood the real science — once I understood that true healing happens in the empty spaces — everything shifted. Hunger became strength. Rest became strategy. Fasting became a secret weapon. It's important to do it safely, and it's important to listen to your body. But the bottom line is simple: Cancer loves an environment of constant feeding and inflammation. Fasting flips the environment against cancer — and back in your favor. If you're facing cancer, or trying to rebuild your health, I can tell you firsthand: Fasting is one of the greatest tools you can add to your arsenal. Not to punish your body. Not to weaken yourself. But to give your body the break it desperately needs to fight back — and win.

Chapter 6

Welcome to Your New Life (And New Food)

Change is never easy. But sometimes life gives you no choice. After my diagnosis, after everything I learned about what fuels cancer and what heals the body, I realized one simple truth: If I wanted a new outcome, I had to build a new life. Not just a few tweaks. Not just cutting out a few "bad foods." I had to rebuild from the ground up — body, mind, and spirit. And one of the biggest changes started with the food on my plate. For most of my life, I ate like most people do. Whatever was easy. Whatever tasted good. Whatever filled me up after a long day's work. I thought I was strong enough to handle anything. But strength isn't about how much you can carry — it's about knowing when to put things down that are hurting you. Cancer forced me to look at food through a whole new lens: What feeds cancer? What starves it? What rebuilds healthy cells? What strengthens the immune system? I realized that every bite could either feed the problem or fuel the solution. That's when my new life — and my new way of eating — truly began. I swapped processed foods for real, whole foods.

I chose meals that were clean, anti-inflammatory, and packed with healing power. I prioritized vegetables, berries, clean proteins, healthy fats, and powerful healing herbs like turmeric and black pepper. I didn't just eat to survive. I ate to heal. And something incredible happened: My energy came back. My body handled chemotherapy better than anyone expected. My mind became clearer. My spirit became stronger.

I realized that healing wasn't about punishment. It wasn't about restriction.

It was about feeding my body what it was truly crying out for all along. Was it easy? No. Was it worth it? Absolutely. If you're reading this, you might be at the same crossroads. A place where the old ways have to be left behind — not because they were all bad, but because they no longer serve the life you're building now.

This isn't about perfection. It's about direction. Every better choice you make is a step toward a stronger, healthier, more powerful you. Welcome to your new life. A life where food is not the enemy. A life where every meal becomes an act of healing. A life where you take your power back, one bite at a time.

Chapter 7

Foods to Pause (Even If They're Healthy)

Before my diagnosis, if you had asked anyone around me, they would have said I was one of the healthiest people they knew. I didn't smoke. I hadn't touched alcohol for over six years. I ate salads regularly. I drank green tea every day. I had berries with honey and cinnamon for breakfast — what could be healthier than that? People even used to joke that I was a bit of a "health freak." And yet... cancer still found its way into my body. Looking back with clearer eyes, I can see things differently now. I did a lot right. But there was one hidden weakness that slipped through the cracks: Sugar. I had a real sweet tooth — and, if I'm honest, there was probably some form of refined sugar in my body almost every single day of my life. It wasn't always obvious. It wasn't just about eating chocolate bars or desserts. Sugar hides in so many "normal" foods — sauces, breads, snacks — and even in "healthy" foods when you don't realize how much natural sugar is stacking up. The berries and honey I loved were good — but they also kept my blood sugar higher than it needed to be. And cancer loves sugar. Cancer cells are greedy. They need massive amounts of glucose (sugar) to grow, multiply, and spread. Every spike of blood sugar gives cancer cells more fuel to survive and thrive. That's why, when you're fighting cancer, it's not enough to just eat "healthy." You have to eat strategically. That means being willing to pause even some foods that are normally considered healthy — at least while your body is in full healing mode.

Foods I had to rethink and pause included: Honey (natural, but very high in sugar) Large servings of fruit (especially very sweet fruits like bananas, grapes, mangoes) Packaged "health" snacks (often loaded with hidden sugars) Certain grains and breads (even wholegrain — they can spike blood sugar) It wasn't about demonizing these foods forever.

It was about giving my body the cleanest possible environment to heal — without constantly feeding the disease I was trying to beat. Once I understood that, my entire relationship with food changed. Now, when I eat berries, it's in small amounts — and without honey. Now, when I choose salads, I watch for hidden sugars in dressings.

Now, I build every meal thinking: "Does this fuel me — or does it fuel the cancer?" The truth is, even healthy foods can be misused if we're not looking closely. And when you're fighting for your life, you have to be willing to look closer than you ever have before.

Chapter 8

Cancer's Favorite Foods

If cancer had a shopping list, it wouldn't be filled with cigarettes and alcohol — it would be full of everyday foods found in most people's kitchens. That's what shocked me the most. I didn't smoke. I hadn't drunk alcohol for years. I thought I ate well. But once I started digging into what cancer actually feeds on, I realised I'd been unknowingly helping it thrive. Cancer is a metabolic disease at its core and it's fueled by what's in your bloodstream. And if there's one thing it absolutely loves, it's sugar. Not just the white stuff in desserts I'm talking about: Hidden sugars in sauces, cereals, muesli bars "Healthy" sugars like honey, agave, maple syrup Refined carbohydrates that quickly turn into sugar in the body (white bread, pastries, pasta) Glucose is cancer's favourite food. The more your blood sugar spikes, the more fuel you give it to grow and spread. And it's not just sugar cancer also thrives in inflammatory environments, especially when fed by: Vegetable and seed oils (canola, sunflower, soybean) Processed meats (bacon, ham, sausages with preservatives) Highly refined flours and snack foods, Artificial sweeteners and additives. When I look back, I realise I'd probably had refined sugar in my body nearly every day of my life.

That constant drip of sugar and inflammation was like adding petrol to a slow-burning fire. Even some of the things I thought were healthy like store-bought sauces, wraps, crackers — were secretly loaded with ingredients that made things worse. I didn't know. No one ever told me. And I wasn't alone. These foods are everywhere — marketed as normal, even "wholesome." But they create an internal environment where cancer cells can thrive and multiply. The moment I learned this, everything changed. I stopped asking, "Is this food healthy?" I started asking, "Is this food going to help me beat cancer — or feed it?" That one question became my compass.

When I started removing cancer's favourite foods, my body started changing: Inflammation dropped, Energy returned, my recovery improved, I felt cleaner, lighter, stronger And the best part? I wasn't starving myself.

I was just cutting off the fuel supply to what was trying to destroy me.

If you're fighting cancer, this might be one of the most important chapters in this whole book. Because you can be doing everything else right — taking the meds, fasting, exercising — but if you're still feeding the enemy, you're slowing your own healing down. When you take away the foods cancer loves, you take back the power.

Chapter 9

Why Food Can Kill Cancer

Once I stripped out the foods that were feeding cancer, the next question I asked was: "What can I eat to fight it?" That question changed everything. Because food isn't just fuel. Food is chemistry. Every bite you take sends messages to your cells — messages to either fight or fold. And it turns out, nature has already given us an entire toolbox of anti-cancer weapons — right in the form of whole, healing food. When I started studying the science, I discovered that certain foods don't just "support" the body... they actively work against cancer.

Some starve cancer cells by cutting off their fuel supply.

Some trigger cell death (apoptosis) in damaged or mutated cells.

Some block angiogenesis — the process that cancer uses to build blood vessels and grow.

Others boost your immune system, so your body can do what it was designed to do: identify and destroy the threat

The more I learned, the more I saw food as medicine — real, measurable, and powerful.

Here are just a few examples:

Broccoli, cauliflower, and Brussels sprouts — rich in sulforaphane, known to help neutralize carcinogens and boost detox

Turmeric with black pepper — a powerful anti-inflammatory

combination that can reduce tumour-promoting pathways

Garlic and onions — loaded with sulphur compounds that enhance immune activity and may suppress tumour growth

Green tea — packed with catechins (like EGCG) that have shown anti-cancer properties in studies

Berries — rich in antioxidants and compounds that protect DNA from damage.

This wasn't about eating "clean" for the sake of it. This was about targeted nutrition eating with intention, eating to win. I started loading my meals with these foods every day. They became my frontline soldiers — not in a war of fear, but in a strategy of healing.

And the best part? This isn't just about fighting cancer.

These same foods also: Reduce inflammation, Improve digestion Support detox pathways to Enhance energy, mood, and recovery In a world full of pills, procedures, and high-tech machines, it's easy to forget the power sitting on your plate.

But I'm here to tell you: Food can kill cancer. Not with magic. Not with hype.

But with consistent, daily choices that shift your entire internal environment.

You don't have to understand every molecule to know this: When you eat real, living food — food designed by nature — you give your body the tools to fight back. Every healing meal you eat is like casting a vote — not just against cancer, but for life.

I didn't learn all this overnight — and I didn't do it alone. I used ChatGPT almost every day as a simple, powerful tool to help guide my decisions. I'd ask things like:

Is this vegetable safe during chemotherapy?
What are the benefits of turmeric and black pepper?
Does this ingredient feed or fight cancer?

It saved me hours of digging — and gave me instant, clear answers when I needed them most. If you're going through this journey, don't carry the research burden alone. Open ChatGPT, ask what you need to know, and start learning faster. It helped me build this new way of eating — and it can help you too.

Chapter 10

The Anti-Cancer Vegetable List

When I started looking at food as medicine, I realized that not all vegetables are equal. Some aren't just "healthy" — they're powerful tools that help your body detox, lower inflammation, and even fight cancer directly. I wanted to know: "Which vegetables are the strongest cancer-fighters?" I used ChatGPT as a quick research partner. I'd ask, "What's in this vegetable that helps fight cancer?" or "Is this safe to eat during chemotherapy?" It saved me hours — and gave me confidence that the foods I was choosing were really helping me. Over time, I built this list:

✅ Broccoli

Contains sulforaphane, known to help neutralize carcinogens and boost detox

✅ **Cauliflower**

Supports liver detox and reduces inflammation

✅ **Brussels sprouts**

Rich in glucosinolates, helping block cancer development

✅ **Kale**

High in antioxidants, vitamins A, C, K, plus anti-cancer compounds

✅ **Spinach**

Packed with chlorophyll, folate, and cancer-protective carotenoids

✅ **Garlic**

Contains allicin, boosting immune function and helping reduce tumor growth

✅ **Onions**

Loaded with quercetin and Sulphur compounds that enhance detox pathways

✅ **Leeks**

Similar benefits to garlic and onions; supports digestion and immunity

✅ **Cabbage**

A simple, inexpensive cruciferous vegetable with anti-cancer properties

✅ **Carrots**

High in beta-carotene and other antioxidants

✅ **Beetroot**

Supports liver detox and contains anti-inflammatory betalains

✅ **Mushrooms**

(shiitake, maitake, reishi) Immune-boosting and anti-tumor effects I made sure these vegetables became the foundation of my meals.

Whether it was sautéed spinach in my omelette, steamed broccoli and cauliflower with dinner, or adding garlic and onions to nearly every dish — these foods weren't just "good for me."

They were part of my healing team.

The great thing is, they're easy to find, easy to prepare, and can be rotated daily so you don't get bored.

If you're fighting cancer, recovering, or just trying to protect your health — start here. You don't need to complicate it. You don't need fancy superfoods from far away.

Just real vegetables, packed with natural compounds designed by nature to protect you.

And if you're ever unsure, do what I did — ask ChatGPT about a vegetable before you eat it. It takes 30 seconds, and it gives you confidence you're feeding your body, not the problem.

Chapter 11

The Anti-Cancer Fruit List

Just like vegetables, some fruits go beyond being "healthy" they contain compounds that actively protect your cells and support healing. After I learned how much cancer loves sugar, I knew I had to be careful with fruit. I didn't want to give cancer the sugar it craved. But I didn't want to miss out on the powerful anticancer benefits that certain fruits carry. That's when I used ChatGPT to help me dig deeper. I'd ask: "Does this fruit have anti-cancer properties?" "Is this fruit high or low in sugar?" "Is this safe to eat during chemo?" It gave me quick answers, saving me hours of digging through conflicting advice online. Over time, I built this trusted list of fruits I used regularly — safe, powerful, and part of my healing:

✓ **Blueberries**
Rich in anthocyanins, powerful antioxidants that protect DNA and reduce tumor growth

✓ **Blackberries**
High in polyphenols and fiber, supporting detox and gut health

✓ **Raspberries**
Contain ellagic acid, linked to cancer cell suppression

✓ **Strawberries**
Good source of vitamin C and flavonoids

✓ **Cranberries**
(unsweetened)

Anti-inflammatory and supports urinary tract health

✅ **Pomegranate seeds**

Contain punicalagins, shown to slow cancer cell growth in studies

✅ **Avocado**

High in healthy fats, carotenoids, and anti-inflammatory properties

✅ **Lemon and lime**

Alkalizing, immune-boosting, rich in vitamin C

✅ **Papaya**

Contains papain, which aids digestion and may support immunity.

I made these fruits part of my daily plan — but always in moderation.

I didn't pile them into big smoothies or bowls.

I'd have a small handful of berries, maybe a few slices of pomegranate, or add lemon to my water.

This way, I still got the powerful compounds without flooding my system with excess sugar.

That's what I want you to remember: Even with fruit, it's not "the more, the better" — it's "the right amount, at the right time."

And if I was ever unsure, I'd ask ChatGPT: "How much of this fruit is safe while fighting cancer?" It's one of the easiest ways to get clear answers without spending hours trying to figure it out. You don't have to fear fruit. But you do have to respect how cancer uses sugar. This list gave me peace of mind — and I hope it gives you the same.

Chapter 12

Recipes to Kill Cancer

Throughout my journey, I discovered that food could be a powerful ally in healing. By focusing on nutrient-dense, anti-inflammatory meals, I aimed to nourish my body and support its natural defenses. The following daily meal plan outlines the core meals that became staples in my routine.

My Daily Healing Meal Plan Breakfast:

Healing Omelette: Free-range eggs, baby spinach, mushrooms, goat's cheese (pasteurized), capsicum, turmeric, black pepper, and olive oil.

Post-Meal Snack (3 times a day):

My Power Bar: Homemade bars packed with oats, nut butter, coconut oil, seeds, cacao, turmeric, cinnamon, and mixed nuts.

Afternoon Snack:

Sardines or mackerel (wild-caught) with avocado and tomato, seasoned with turmeric, black pepper, and tamari soy sauce.

Dinner Options:

Steamed broccoli, Brussels sprouts, wild-caught fish, and sweet potato. Cancer-fighting Bolognese served with Brussels sprouts or gluten-free pasta.
Fresh salad with grilled fish, seasoned with mixed herbs, turmeric, black pepper, garlic, and ginger.

These meals formed the foundation of my healing — they weren't just healthy; they were intentional, built to support my body's fight against cancer.

Detailed Recipes

1. **Healing Omelette**

Ingredients:

3 free-range eggs Handful of baby spinach

½ cup mushrooms, sliced

sprinkle of soft goat's cheese (pasteurized)

½ capsicum, diced

¼ tsp turmeric powder black pepper

1 tbsp olive oil

Instructions:

In a bowl, whisk the eggs with turmeric and black pepper. Heat olive oil in a pan over medium heat. Sauté mushrooms and capsicum until tender. Add spinach and cook until wilted. Put to the side.
Pour in the egg mixture and cook until the omelette is set. Add mushrooms, spinach and capsicum, Sprinkle goat's cheese on top, fold the omelette, and serve warm.

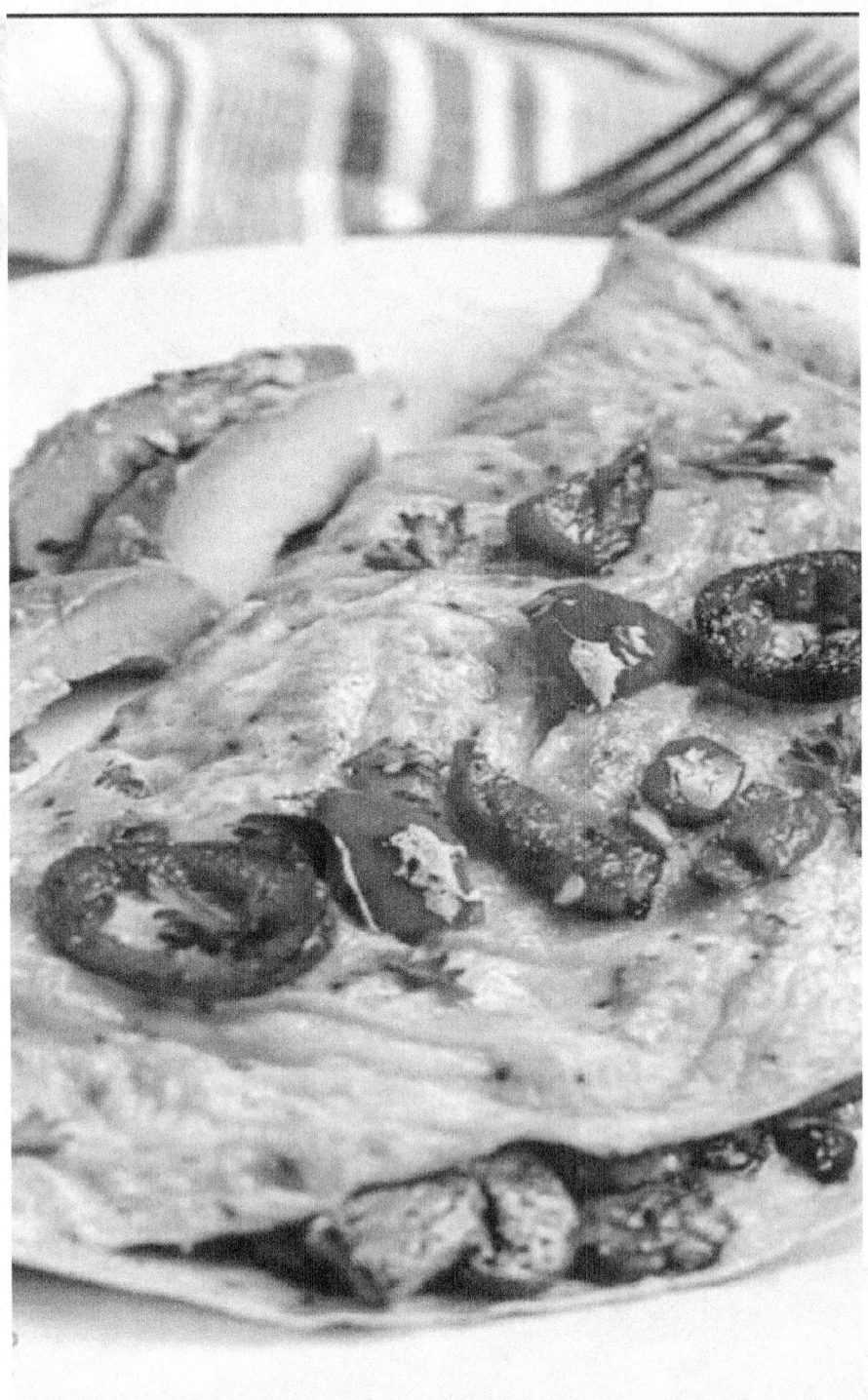

2. My Power Bar

Ingredients:

2 cups rolled oats (gluten-free if needed)

½ cup nut butter (almond, peanut, or cashew)

¼ cup coconut oil, melted

2 tbsp raw cacao powder

1 tsp turmeric powder

Black pepper

½ tsp organic vanilla extract

½ tsp ground cinnamon

1 cup frozen berries

1 cup of mixed nuts

2 tbsp chia seeds

1 tbsp flaxseed

1 tbsp ground hemp seed

1 tbsp honey

2 chopped dates

Instructions:

In a large bowl,
mix melted coconut oil, nut butter, honey, dates and vanilla extract until smooth. Add all other ingredients in the bowl, mix well and combine. pour the wet mixture into a rubber mold and press firmly into it.

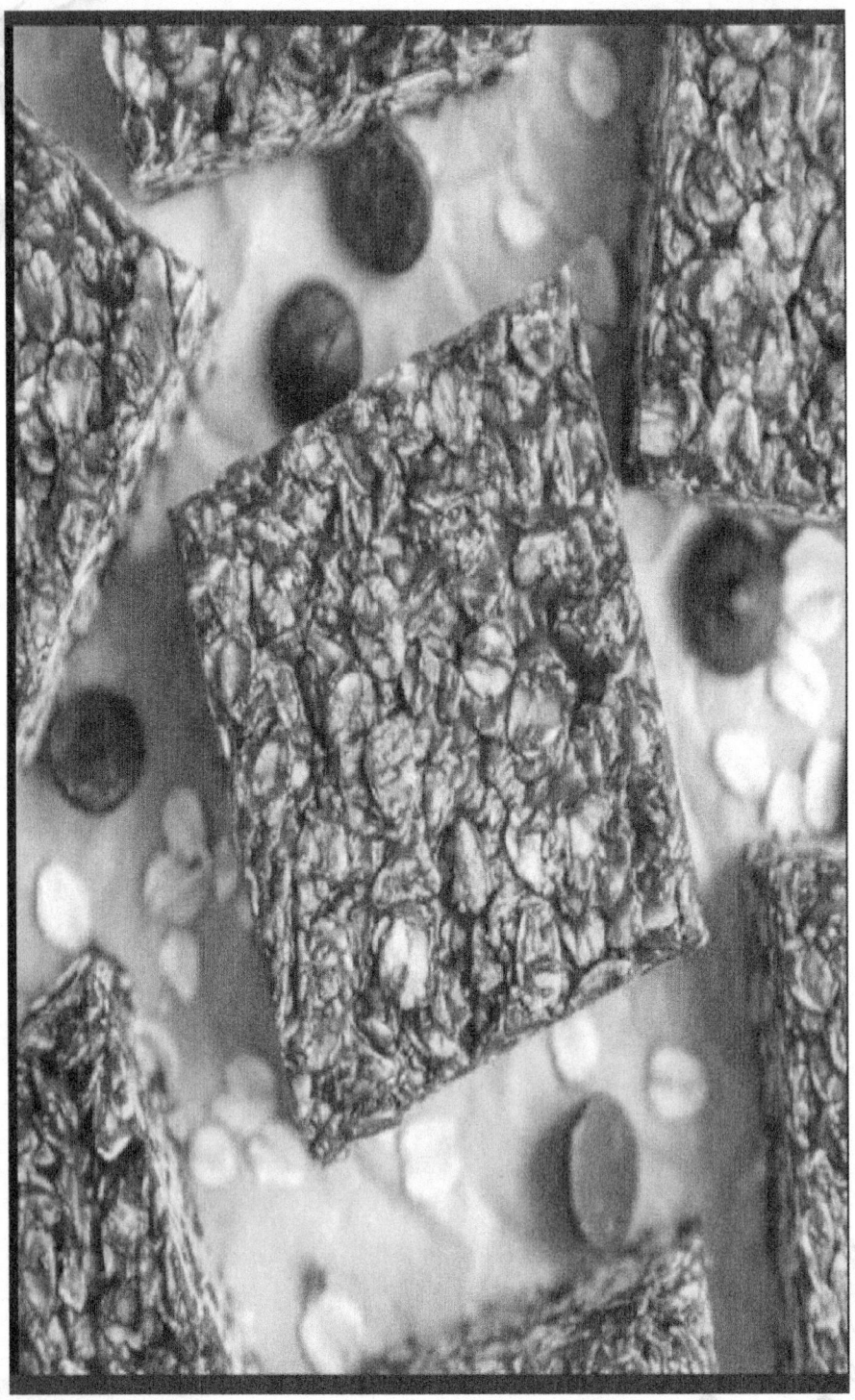

Place in the freezer for at least 1 hour until set. Store bars in the fridge or freezer.

3. Sardines or Mackerel with Avocado and Tomato

Ingredients:

1 can sardines or mackerel (wild-caught)
1 ripe avocado, sliced
1 tomato, diced
¼ tsp turmeric powder
Pinch of black pepper
1 tsp tamari soy sauce

Instructions:

Arrange avocado slices and diced tomato on a plate.
Top with sardines or mackerel.
Sprinkle turmeric and black pepper over the top.
Drizzle with tamari soy sauce and serve.

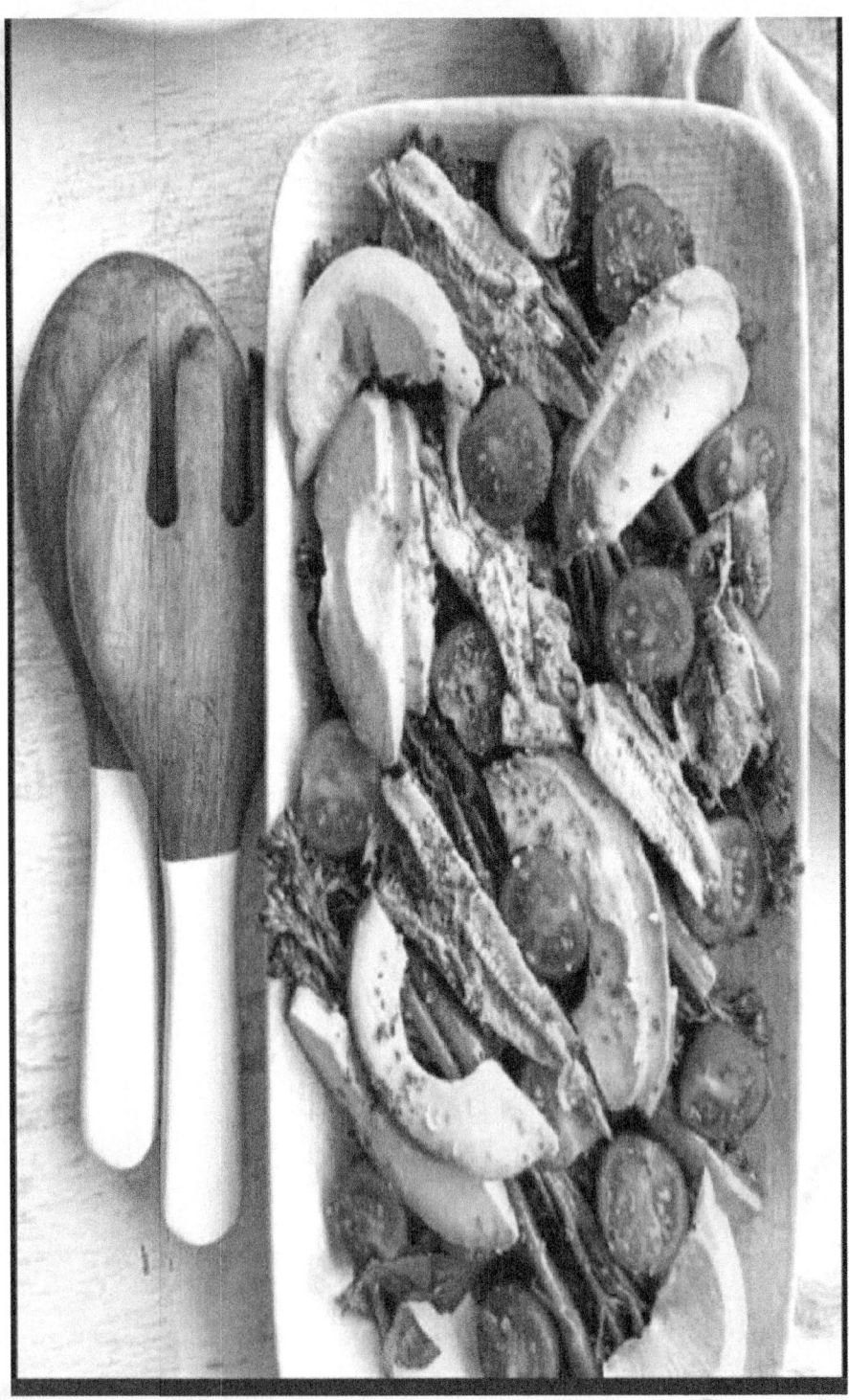

4. Steamed Broccoli, Brussels Sprouts, Wild-Caught Fish, and Sweet Potato

Ingredients:

1 cup broccoli florets

1 cup Brussels sprouts,

halved 1 fillet wild-caught fish (e.g., barramundi)

1 medium sweet potato, sliced

1 tbsp olive oil

¼ tsp turmeric powder

Pinch of black pepper

1 clove garlic, minced

1 tsp grated ginger

Instructions:

Steam broccoli and Brussels sprouts until tender.
Bake sweet potato slices at 200°C (400°F) for 20 minutes or until soft.
Season fish with turmeric, black pepper, garlic, and ginger.
Pan-fry fish in olive oil over medium heat until cooked through. Serve fish alongside steamed vegetables and sweet potato.

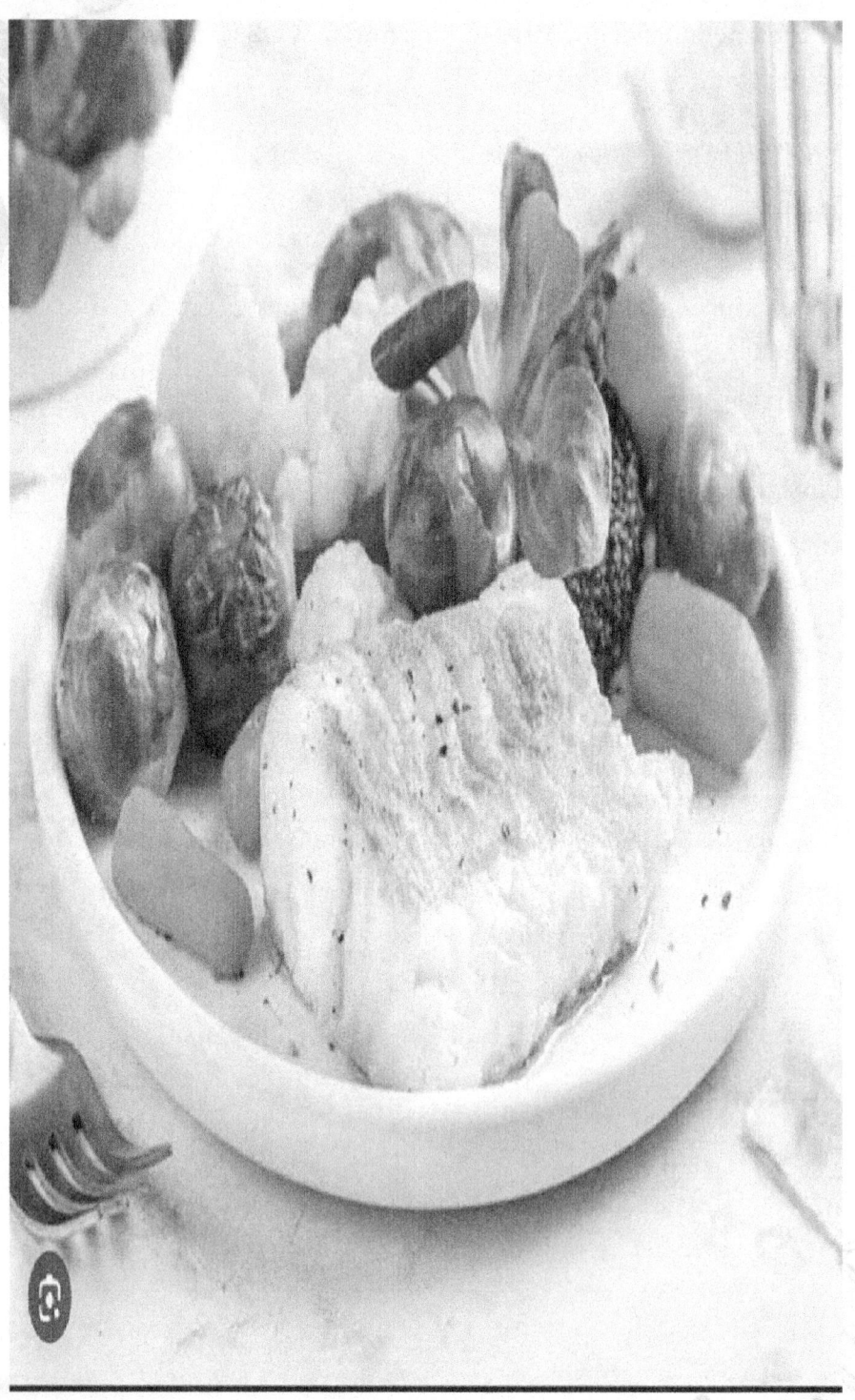

5. Cancer-Fighting Bolognese

Ingredients:

500g turkey mince or grass-fed beef
1 onion, diced
2 cloves garlic, minced
1 capsicum, diced
1 tbsp olive oil
1 tsp turmeric powder
½ tsp black pepper
1 tsp dried oregano 400g can organic chopped tomatoes (no added sugar)
2 cups spinach leaves Brussels sprouts or gluten-free pasta, for serving

Instructions:

Heat olive oil in a pan over medium heat.
Sauté onion, garlic, and capsicum until softened.
Add mince and cook until browned.
Stir in turmeric, black pepper, and oregano.
Pour in chopped tomatoes and simmer for 15 minutes.
Add spinach and cook until wilted.
Serve over steamed Brussels sprouts or gluten-free pasta.

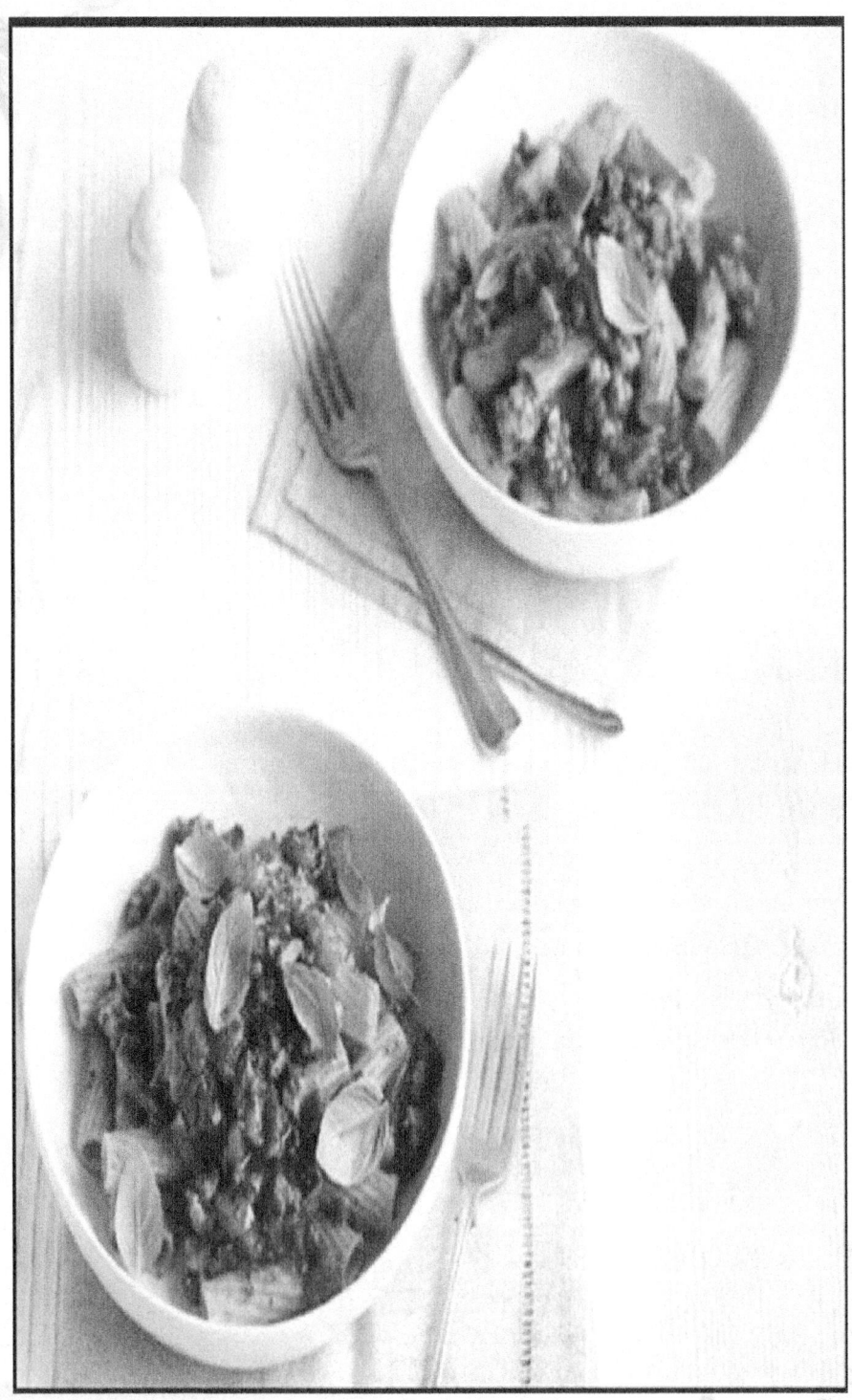

6. Fresh Salad with Grilled Fish 1 fillet wild-caught fish (e.g., barramundi)

Ingredients:

Mixed salad greens
1 tomato, sliced
½ cucumber, sliced
¼ red onion, thinly sliced
1 tbsp olive oil
¼ tsp turmeric powder
Pinch of black pepper
1 clove garlic, minced
1 tsp grated ginger
1 tsp mixed herbs

Instructions:

Season fish with turmeric, black pepper, garlic, ginger, and mixed herbs. Grill fish until cooked through.
In a bowl, combine salad greens, tomato, cucumber, and red onion. Drizzle with olive oil and toss to combine.
Top salad with grilled fish and serve.

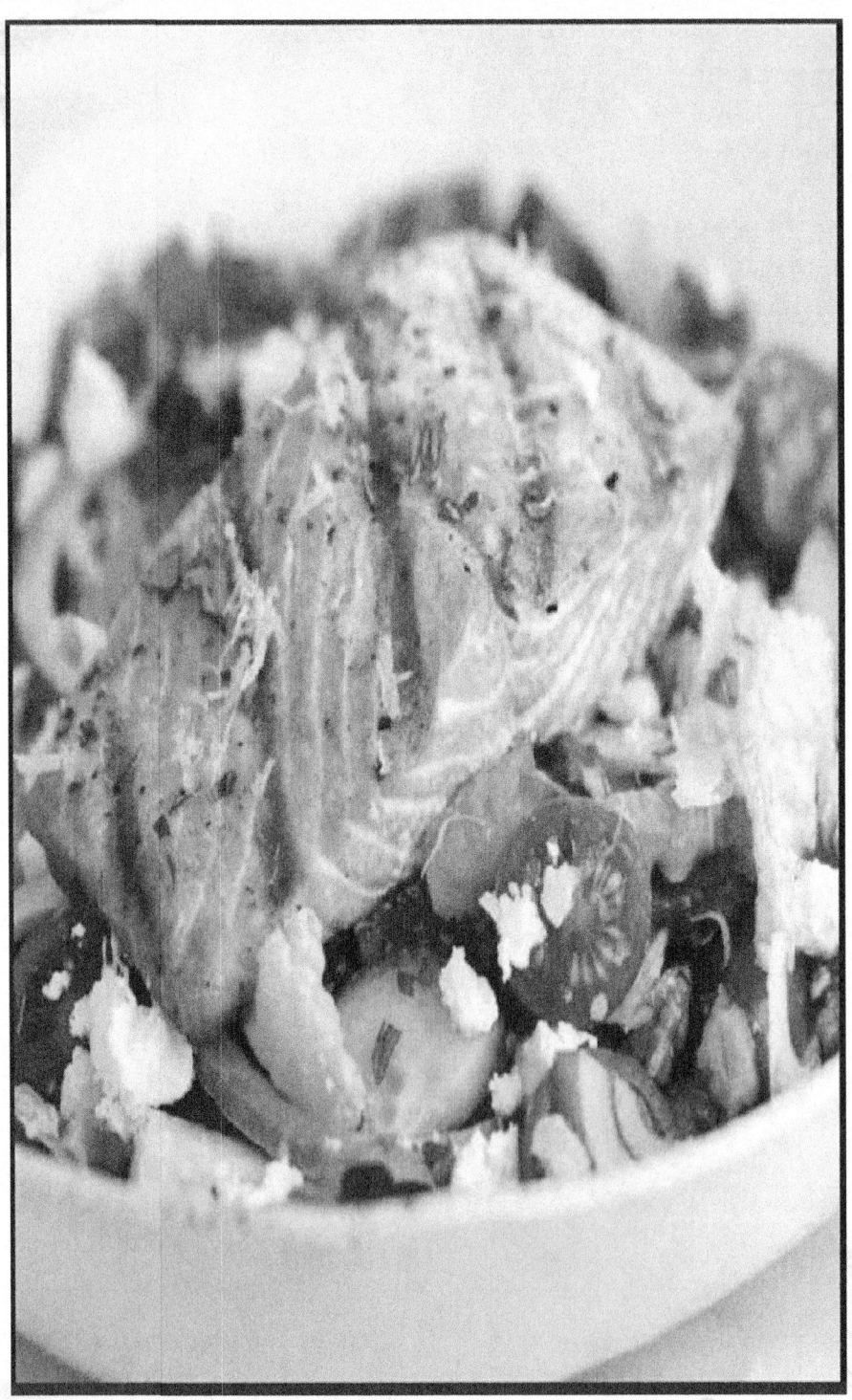

Expanding Recipes for Readers

I want this book to give readers plenty of variety, not just my core meals. I'll be adding:

More breakfast options

More snacks and light meals

More hearty dinner recipes

Soups, stews, broths

Smoothies, drinks, sauces

Healing desserts (low-sugar, cancer-friendly)

The goal is to give every reader a practical, flexible meal plan no matter their tastes or preferences, while keeping every recipe aligned with the anti-cancer principles I used. These recipes were more than just meals; they were a testament to the power of intentional eating. Each dish was crafted to support my body's healing process,

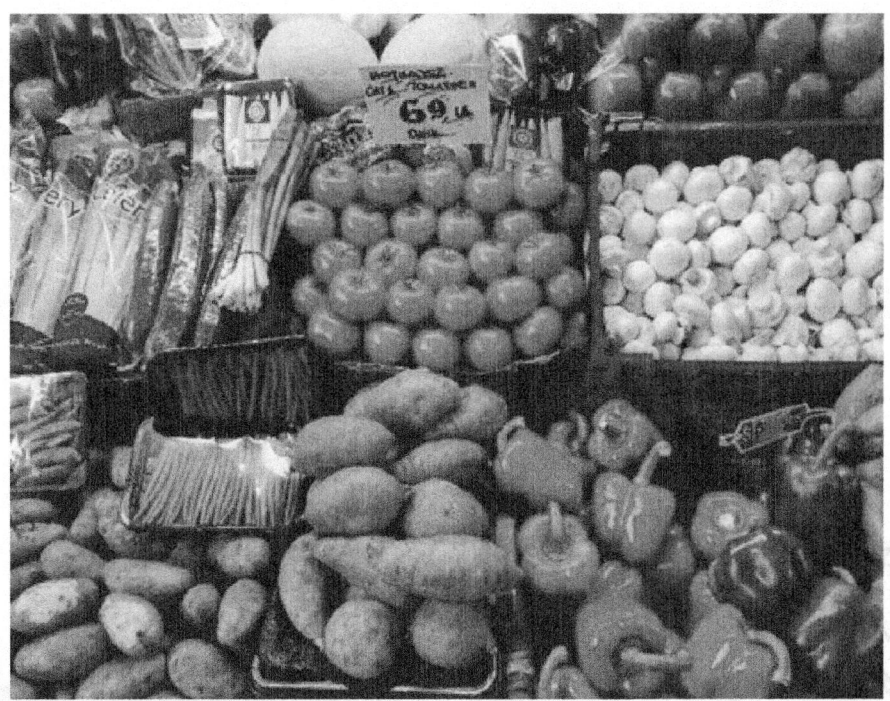

Healing Recipes for Readers
Breakfast Options
1. Sweet Potato Breakfast Hash

Ingredients:

1 small sweet potato, peeled and diced
¼ small red onion, diced
½ capsicum, diced
3–4 mushrooms, sliced
Handful baby spinach
1 clove garlic, minced
Olive oil for cooking
Sea salt, black pepper, pinch of turmeric

Instructions:

Heat olive oil in a skillet over medium heat.
Add sweet potato and cook for 8–10 minutes until softened, stirring occasionally. Add onion, capsicum, mushrooms, and garlic; sauté for another 3–4 minutes.
Stir in spinach, turmeric, salt, and pepper; cook 1–2 minutes until spinach wilts. Serve warm as a hearty, veggie-packed breakfast.

2. Avocado & Tomato on Gluten-Free Toast

Ingredients:

1 slice gluten-free bread
½ ripe avocado
1 small tomato, sliced
1 tsp lemon juice Black pepper and oregano

Instructions:

Toast the gluten-free bread to your liking.

In a bowl, mash the avocado with lemon juice and black pepper. Spread mashed avocado over the toast.

Top with tomato slices and a sprinkle of oregano. Serve immediately.

3. Berry & Nut Smoothie

Ingredients:

1 cup frozen mixed berries
1 cup unsweetened almond milk 1 tbsp almond butter
1 tbsp chia seeds
½ tsp turmeric Dash of black pepper

Instructions:

Add all ingredients to a blender.

Blend on high until smooth and creamy.

Pour into a glass and enjoy immediately.

4. Turmeric Baked Beans on Toast

Ingredients:

1 cup organic canned mixed beans (or baked beans)
1 clove garlic, minced
½ tsp turmeric Dash of black pepper
½ cup chopped tomatoes (fresh or canned)
Olive oil for cooking
1 slice gluten-free bread

Instructions:

Heat olive oil in a small pan.
Add garlic and sauté for 1 minute.
Add tomatoes, turmeric, and black pepper; cook for 3 minutes. Stir in beans and simmer for 5 minutes until heated through.
Toast gluten-free bread and serve beans on top.

5. Healing Green Smoothie
Ingredients:
1 cup baby spinach
½ cup frozen mango
½ banana
1 tbsp ground flaxseed
1 tsp spirulina or greens powder (optional) 1 cup unsweetened almond milk

Instructions:
Add all ingredients to a blender. Blend until smooth and creamy. Pour into a glass and serve.

6. Cancer-Fighting Chia Pudding
Ingredients:
3 tbsp chia seeds
1 cup unsweetened almond milk
½ cup blueberries
1 tbsp chopped walnuts 1 tbsp coconut flakes
1 tsp tahini

Instructions:

In a jar or bowl, mix chia seeds and almond milk.
Stir well. Refrigerate overnight or for at least 4 hours to thicken.
Before serving, top with blueberries, walnuts, coconut flakes, and drizzle tahini on top.

7. Mushroom & Spinach Scramble

Ingredients:

2 eggs
3–4 mushrooms, sliced
Handful of baby spinach
1 clove garlic, minced
½ tsp turmeric Dash of black pepper
Olive oil for cooking

Instructions:

Heat olive oil in a pan over medium heat. Add garlic and mushrooms; cook for 3–4 minutes until mushrooms soften. Add spinach and cook for 1 minute until wilted.
Beat eggs in a bowl with turmeric, black pepper, and a pinch of salt.
Pour eggs into the pan and scramble until cooked through.
Serve warm.

8. Buckwheat Pancakes
Ingredients:

½ cup buckwheat flour
½ tsp baking powder
½ tsp cinnamon 1 egg
½ cup unsweetened almond milk Coconut oil for cooking

Mixed berries for topping Coconut yogurt (optional)

Instructions:

In a bowl, mix buckwheat flour, baking powder, and cinnamon. Add egg and almond milk; whisk to a smooth batter.
Heat a small amount of coconut oil in a pan over medium heat. Pour in batter to form small pancakes;
cook 2–3 minutes each side until golden.
Serve topped with berries and a spoonful of coconut yogurt.

9. Quinoa Porridge
Ingredients:
½ cup cooked quinoa
1 cup unsweetened almond milk
½ tsp cinnamon
1 small apple, chopped
1 tbsp walnuts
1 tbsp pumpkin seeds

Instructions:

Add cooked quinoa, almond milk, and cinnamon to a small pot. Simmer gently for 5–7 minutes until warm and creamy.
Pour into a bowl; top with chopped apple, walnuts, and pumpkin seeds.

10. Banana & Walnut Buckwheat Porridge
Ingredients:
½ cup buckwheat groats (soaked overnight & rinsed)
1 cup unsweetened almond milk
½ banana, sliced
1 tbsp chopped walnuts

½ tsp cinnamon

1 tsp flaxseed Optional: drizzle of tahini

Instructions:

In a small pot, combine soaked buckwheat and almond milk.
Bring to a gentle simmer; cook for 7–10 minutes until soft and creamy.
Stir in cinnamon and flaxseed.
Serve topped with banana slices, walnuts, and an optional drizzle of tahini.

Snack & Light Meal Options

1. Avocado Rice Cakes

Ingredients:

1–2 brown rice cakes (unsalted)
½ ripe avocado
1 tsp lemon juice
Sea salt, black pepper Optional:
sliced cherry tomatoes or radish

Instructions:

Mash avocado with lemon juice, salt, and pepper.
Spread on rice cakes.
Top with tomatoes or radish if desired.

2. Turmeric Hummus with Veggie Sticks

Ingredients:

1 can organic chickpeas, drained and rinsed
1 tbsp tahini
1 tbsp olive oil
Juice of ½ lemon

1 small garlic clove
½ tsp turmeric, pinch of black pepper
Water as needed

Instructions:

Blend all ingredients in a food processor until smooth.
Add water 1 tbsp at a time for desired consistency.
Serve with sticks of carrot, cucumber, or celery.

3. Goat's Cheese & Tomato Stuffed Mushrooms

Ingredients:

4 large button mushrooms
2 tbsp soft goat's cheese
4 cherry tomatoes, chopped
Pinch of oregano

Instructions:

Preheat oven to 180°C. Remove mushroom stems, place on a baking tray.
Mix goat's cheese and tomatoes;
fill mushroom caps.
Sprinkle with oregano and bake for 12–15 minutes.

4. Berry & Nut Yogurt Cup

Ingredients:

½ cup Greek or coconut yogurt (unsweetened, full-fat)
¼ cup mixed berries
1 tbsp chopped walnuts or almonds Dash of cinnamon

Instructions:

Layer yogurt, berries, and nuts in a small bowl or jar. Sprinkle with cinnamon and enjoy chilled.

5. Roasted Chickpeas (Savory Crunch)

Ingredients:

1 can chickpeas, drained and dried
1 tbsp olive oil
½ tsp turmeric
½ tsp smoked paprika
Pinch of sea salt

Instructions:

Preheat oven to 200°C. Toss chickpeas with oil and spices. Spread on tray and roast 25–30 mins until crispy.

6. Mashed Avocado & Tuna Cups

Ingredients:

½ avocado
½ tin wild-caught tuna (in spring water), drained
1 tsp lemon juice Pinch of sea salt Optional: chopped parsley

Instructions:

Mix all ingredients in a bowl.
Scoop into small lettuce cups or cucumber slices.

7. Oat & Seed Crackers
Ingredients:

½ cup oats

¼ cup ground flaxseed
¼ cup sunflower seeds
¼ cup water Pinch of sea salt

Instructions:

Mix all ingredients; let sit 10 mins.

Spread thinly on baking paper.

Bake at 160°C for 25 mins or until crisp.

Cool and break into crackers.

8. Cucumber & Hummus Bites

Ingredients:

½ cucumber, sliced

½ cup hummus (see recipe above or store-bought)

Paprika or turmeric for garnish

Instructions:

Top each cucumber slice with 1 tsp hummus.

Dust with paprika or turmeric for flavour and colour.

9. Almond Date Energy Balls

Ingredients:

1 cup almonds

6 pitted Medjool dates 1 tbsp cacao powder

½ tsp cinnamon

1 tbsp coconut oil

Instructions:

Blend all ingredients in a food processor until sticky.

Roll into small balls and chill in fridge for 1 hour.

10. Pumpkin Seed Pâté with Crackers or Veggies

Ingredients:

½ cup raw pumpkin seeds (pepitas)

1 tbsp olive oil

Juice of ½ lemon

1 small garlic clove

Pinch of turmeric and black pepper

2 tbsp water (more as needed)

Optional: chopped parsley or dill for garnish

Instructions:

Lightly toast pumpkin seeds in a dry pan for 3–5 minutes, stirring until they begin to pop.

Let cool. Add seeds, garlic, lemon juice, olive oil, turmeric, pepper, and water to a blender or food processor.

Blend until smooth, scraping down sides and adding a splash more water if needed.

Serve chilled with oat & seed crackers, cucumber slices, or celery sticks.

Soups (5 Recipes)

1. Immune-Boosting Mushroom & Garlic Soup

Ingredients:

1 tbsp olive oil

1 small onion, chopped 3 garlic cloves, minced

1 cup shiitake mushrooms, sliced

1 cup white button mushrooms, sliced 1 tsp thyme

1 tsp turmeric, pinch of black pepper 3 cups vegetable broth

Handful baby spinach (added at end)

Instructions:

Heat olive oil in a pot. Sauté onion and garlic until soft.
Add mushrooms, thyme, turmeric, and pepper.
Cook 5–7 mins.
Add broth, bring to boil, then simmer for 15 minutes.
Stir in spinach to wilt before serving.

2. Broccoli & Cauliflower Soup

Ingredients:

1 tbsp olive oil
1 small leek or onion, chopped
1 garlic clove
1½ cups broccoli florets
1½ cups cauliflower florets
1 tsp turmeric, pinch of pepper
3 cups veggie stock:
2 tbsp coconut cream for extra smoothness

Instructions:

Sauté leek/onion and garlic in olive oil until soft.
Add broccoli, cauliflower, turmeric, and pepper. Stir well. Pour in stock, simmer 20 mins. Blend until smooth.
Add coconut cream if using.

3. Creamy Pumpkin, Carrot & Ginger Soup

Ingredients:

1 tbsp olive oil
1 cup pumpkin, peeled & diced
1 carrot, chopped
1 small onion

1 tsp grated ginger 1 tsp turmeric

3 cups vegetable stock

Instructions:

Sauté onion and ginger in olive oil until fragrant.

Add pumpkin, carrot, turmeric, and stock.

Simmer until soft (20–25 mins), then blend until smooth.

4. Lentil & Vegetable Soup

Ingredients:

1 tbsp olive oil

1 garlic clove

1 carrot, chopped

1 celery stalk, chopped

½ zucchini, chopped

½ cup red lentils

½ tsp cumin, turmeric

4 cups veggie broth

Instructions:

Sauté garlic and veggies in oil for 5 mins.

Add lentils, spices, and broth.

Bring to a boil, then simmer for 25 mins.

Optional: blend half for a creamy texture.

5. Healing Green Soup

Ingredients:

1 tbsp olive oil

1 leek or small onion, chopped

2 garlic cloves

1 zucchini, chopped 1 cup broccoli florets

1 cup baby spinach

1 tsp lemon juice

3 cups veggie stock

Instructions:

Sauté leek and garlic in oil.

Add zucchini and broccoli.

Cook 5 mins.

Add stock, simmer 15 mins.

Add spinach and lemon juice, blend until smooth.

Smoothies (5 Recipes)

1. Anti-Inflammatory Berry Smoothie

Ingredients:

1 cup frozen mixed berries

1 cup almond milk (unsweetened)

½ tsp turmeric, dash black pepper

1 tbsp chia seeds

1 tbsp almond butter

Instructions:

Blend all ingredients until smooth.

2. Green Gut-Healer Smoothie

Ingredients:

1 cup spinach

½ frozen banana

½ avocado

1 tbsp flaxseed

1 tsp spirulina or greens powder

1 cup almond milk (unsweetened)

Instructions:

Blend until creamy. Adjust texture with extra milk if needed.

3. Coconut Mango Immune Smoothie

Ingredients:

¾ cup frozen mango

½ banana

½ cup coconut yogurt

1 tbsp shredded coconut

½ tsp ginger

¾ cup water or coconut water

Instructions:

Blend everything until smooth and enjoy chilled.

4. Creamy Cacao Recovery Smoothie

Ingredients:

1 tbsp raw cacao powder

1 cup almond milk (unsweetened) 1 Medjool date or ½ banana

1 tbsp tahini or almond butter 1 tbsp hemp seeds

Instructions:

Blend until creamy and satisfying—perfect post-fast or workout.

5. Detox Beetroot & Berry Smoothie

Ingredients:

½ small cooked beetroot

½ cup mixed berries

1 tbsp lemon juice

1 tsp flaxseed

1 cup water or coconut water

Instructions:

Blend until smooth and bright pink. Earthy, sweet, and cleansing.

Dinner Options

1. Turmeric-Crusted Baked Fish with Greens

Ingredients:

1 white fish fillet (flathead, barramundi, or cod)

½ tsp turmeric Pinch of black pepper Sea salt

1 tsp olive oil Lemon wedge (optional)

Instructions:

Preheat oven to 180°C. Rub fish with turmeric, pepper, salt, and olive oil. Bake for 15–18 mins until flaky.

Serve with steamed broccoli, sprouts, and avocado.

2. Mushroom & Greens Stir-Fry

Ingredients:

1 tbsp olive oil

1 cup mushrooms (shiitake & button), sliced

½ zucchini, sliced

1 cup spinach or Bok choy 1 clove garlic, minced Splash of tamari soy sauce

Instructions:

Heat oil in a pan, sauté garlic and mushrooms for 5 mins.

Add zucchini, cook 3 more mins.

Add greens and tamari, stir-fry until wilted.

3. Quinoa & Roasted Veg Bowl

Ingredients:

½ cup cooked quinoa

½ cup roasted sweet potato

½ cup roasted cauliflower

¼ avocado

Handful baby spinach

Tahini drizzle (1 tsp tahini + lemon + water)

Instructions:

Roast sweet potato and cauliflower with olive oil, turmeric, and pepper.
Serve warm over quinoa with spinach, avocado, and tahini drizzle.

4. Cauliflower Mash with Greens & Fish

Ingredients:

1 white fish fillet

½ head cauliflower 1 tbsp olive oil

Steamed broccoli and spinach Garlic, turmeric, salt

Instructions:

Boil cauliflower, then mash with olive oil, garlic, and turmeric.
Bake or pan-sear fish with lemon and pepper.
Serve with mash and steamed greens.

5. Stuffed Capsicums with Lentils

Ingredients:

2 red capsicums, halved and deseeded

1 cup cooked lentils

¼ zucchini, diced

1 small tomato, diced

1 tbsp olive oil

Garlic, turmeric, pepper

Instructions:

Mix lentils, veg, spices, and oil.

Stuff into capsicum halves.

Bake at 180°C for 25–30 mins.

6. Coconut Veggie Curry with Cauliflower Rice

Ingredients:

1 tbsp coconut oil

1 tsp turmeric,

½ tsp cumin

1 clove garlic

½ onion

1 cup mixed vegetables (e.g., zucchini, carrots, broccoli)

½ cup coconut milk

¼ cup water

1 cup cauliflower rice

Instructions:

Sauté garlic and onion in coconut oil.

Add veggies and spices. Stir-fry for 5 mins.

Add coconut milk and water, simmer 15 mins. Steam or lightly sauté cauliflower rice; serve curry on top.

7. Warm Lentil, Spinach & Sweet Potato Salad with Boiled Egg

Ingredients:

1 cup cooked lentils 1 cup baby spinach

¼ red onion, thinly sliced

½ cup roasted or steamed sweet potato, cubed 1 boiled egg, halved

1 tbsp olive oil Juice of ½ lemon Pinch of cumin

Instructions:

Warm lentils and toss with spinach to wilt slightly.
Add onion, sweet potato, oil, lemon juice, and cumin.
Top with the boiled egg halves. Serve warm.

8. Baked Salmon with Steamed Veg

Ingredients:

1 salmon fillet
Sea salt, turmeric, lemon slice
Broccoli, zucchini, and sprouts

Instructions:

Season salmon with turmeric and salt.
Top with lemon slice.
Bake at 180°C for 15 mins.
Serve with lightly steamed vegetables.

9. Zucchini Noodles with Garlic Mushroom Sauce

Ingredients:

2 zucchinis, spiralised
1 tbsp olive oil
2 garlic cloves
1 cup mushrooms, chopped
¼ cup coconut cream
Pinch of pepper

Instructions:

Sauté garlic and mushrooms in oil for 5–7 mins.
Stir in coconut cream and pepper.
Add zucchini noodles and toss gently for 1–2 mins to soften.

10. Sweet Potato, Avocado & Mushroom Plate

Ingredients:

1 small sweet potato, sliced

½ avocado, sliced

3–4 mushrooms, sliced

1 tsp olive oil

Sea salt, turmeric, black pepper

Instructions:

Roast sweet potato slices with turmeric, pepper, and olive oil at 180°C for 25 mins. Sauté mushrooms in a pan for 4–5 mins.
Serve warm sweet potato with sautéed mushrooms and fresh avocado slices.

Stews, Broths, Drinks & Sauces Stews (3 Recipes)

1. Sweet Potato & Lentil Stew

Ingredients:

1 tbsp olive oil

1 small onion, chopped

1 garlic clove

1 carrot, chopped

½ sweet potato, cubed

½ cup red lentils

½ tsp turmeric, cumin, paprika

3 cups veggie broth

Instructions:

Sauté onion and garlic in olive oil.

Add carrot, sweet potato, lentils, and spices.

Stir well. Pour in broth, bring to boil, then simmer for 25–30 mins until soft and thick.

2. Chickpea & Spinach Coconut Stew

Ingredients:

1 tbsp coconut oil
1 garlic clove, minced
½ onion 1 cup canned chickpeas
1 cup spinach
½ zucchini, diced
½ cup coconut milk
½ tsp turmeric and curry powder

Instructions:

Sauté garlic and onion in coconut oil.
Add chickpeas, zucchini, and spices. Cook 5 mins.
Stir in coconut milk and spinach. Simmer 10 mins.

3. Mushroom & Barley Stew

Ingredients:

1 tbsp olive oil
1 cup mushrooms, chopped
1 small onion
1 garlic clove
½ cup pearl barley, rinsed
3 cups veggie stock
Thyme, pepper

Instructions:

Sauté onion, garlic, and mushrooms.
Add barley, thyme, and stock. Simmer 30–40 mins until barley is tender.

Broths (2 Recipes)

1. Healing Vegetable Broth

Ingredients:

1 celery stalk

1 carrot

½ onion Handful parsley

1 garlic clove

½ tsp turmeric Sea salt, black pepper

4 cups water

Instructions:

Chop all veg.
Add to a pot with turmeric and water. Simmer for 45 minutes.
Strain and sip, or use as a base.

2. Bone Broth (Stove or Slow Cooker)

Ingredients:

1–2 marrow bones (beef or chicken) 2 garlic cloves

1 tbsp apple cider vinegar 1 carrot, celery, onion

2L water

Instructions:

Add all ingredients to a pot.Bring to a boil, then simmer for 6–12 hoursStrain and sip warm or refrigerate for later..

Healing Drinks (3 Recipes)

1. David's Electrolyte Water

Ingredients:

1L water (filtered)

Squeeze of lemon

½ tsp sea salt,

Optional: Herbs of Gold magnesium powder

Instructions:

Mix all in a glass bottle. Sip throughout the day.

2. Green Tea with Turmeric & Black Pepper

Ingredients:

1 organic green tea bag

¼ tsp turmeric Pinch of black pepper

Instructions:

Brew tea.
Add turmeric and pepper.
Let steep 3–5 mins. Drink warm throughout the day.

3. Soursop Leaf Tea (Nighttime Calm)

Ingredients:

2–3 dried soursop leaves

1 cup boiling water

Instructions:

Steep leaves in boiling water for 10–15 mins.
Strain and drink before bed.

Sauces & Dressings (3 Recipes)

1. Tahini Lemon Drizzle

Ingredients:

1 tbsp tahini Juice of ½ lemon

2 tbsp olive oil

2 tbsp apple cider vinegar

Pinch of sea salt

Instructions:

Whisk all ingredients together until smooth and creamy. Use as a dressing for bowls, salads, or roasted vegetables.

2. Mushroom Gravy

Ingredients:

1 tbsp olive oil
½ onion
1 cup mushrooms, finely chopped
1 clove garlic
1 tsp tamari
1 cup veggie broth
½ tsp thyme

Instructions:

Sauté onion, garlic, and mushrooms until soft.
Add tamari, thyme, and broth. Simmer 10 mins.
Blend if smoother texture desired.

3. Creamy Garlic Sauce (David's Favourite)

Ingredients:

1 tbsp olive oil
2 garlic cloves, minced
¼ cup coconut cream
½ tsp onion powder Sea salt and black pepper to taste
Optional: splash of lemon juice

Instructions:

Gently sauté minced garlic in olive oil over low heat for 2–3 minutes (don't let it brown).

Add coconut cream and stir in onion powder, salt, and pepper. Let simmer on low for 5 minutes to thicken slightly.

Add a splash of lemon juice before serving.

Use over fish, sweet potato, or steamed greens.

Healing Desserts (5 Recipes)

1. Chilled Coconut & Berry Cups

Ingredients:

½ cup coconut yogurt (unsweetened)

¼ cup frozen mixed berries 1 tbsp chia seeds

½ tsp cinnamon

Optional: crushed walnuts or flaked coconut

Instructions:

Mix coconut yogurt, chia seeds, and cinnamon in a bowl. Fold in frozen berries.

Spoon into small cups or ramekins and chill 20–30 mins. Top with nuts or coconut flakes before serving.

2. Cinnamon Baked Apples with Walnuts

Ingredients:

1 apple, cored and halved

1 tbsp chopped walnuts

½ tsp cinnamon

1 tsp coconut oil

Optional: drizzle of tahini or spoon of coconut yogurt

Instructions:

Preheat oven to 180°C. Place apples in a small baking dish.

Sprinkle with cinnamon and top with walnuts and coconut oil. Bake 20–25 mins until soft.

Serve warm with optional toppings.

3. Avocado Cacao Mousse

Ingredients:

1 ripe avocado

1 tbsp raw cacao powder

1 Medjool date (or ½ banana for smoother texture)

Splash of vanilla extract Dash of cinnamon

Instructions:

Blend all ingredients until smooth and creamy.

Chill for 30 minutes before serving.

Optional: top with a few berries or a sprinkle of cacao nibs.

4. No-Bake Nut & Seed Bites

Ingredients:

½ cup almonds

2 tbsp pumpkin seeds

2 Medjool dates 1 tbsp tahini or nut butter

1 tbsp shredded coconut Pinch of cinnamon

Instructions:

Pulse all ingredients in a food processor until sticky.

Roll into bite-sized balls. Chill in the fridge for 30 mins before serving.

5. Frozen Banana Berry Bites

Ingredients:

1 banana, sliced
¼ cup mixed berries (chopped if large)
1 tbsp almond butter

Instructions:

Place banana slices on a tray lined with baking paper.
Top with a small dollop of almond butter and a berry or two.
Freeze for 1–2 hours until solid.
Eat cold straight from the freezer as a cool treat.

Final Words: A Message from Me to You

If you've made it this far, I want to say thank you—from one human being to another for walking this road with me. Whether you're reading this as a patient, a carer, or someone simply trying to make better choices, I hope these pages have offered you more than just recipes. I hope they've offered you hope, direction, and a little peace. I didn't set out to become an expert. I was just a bloke trying to get well, trying to keep my head above water after being told I had cancer. But through research, faith, and a relentless drive to give myself the best chance, I built this plan—and it's working. This book isn't about magic cures or silver bullets. It's about giving your body the support it needs to fight, repair, and rise again. It's about giving you control when things feel out of control. I've kept this book short on purpose—because when you're unwell, overwhelmed, or exhausted, the last thing you want is a thick manual. You want something you can trust. Something real. Something that works. If you want to go deeper into my journey— how I handled the diagnosis, what I did each day, and how I stayed strong for my family—you can read the companion book,

[Unstoppable: My fight to live], where I share everything else that helped me keep going. Until then, just know this: You're not alone. You're stronger than you think. And healing is always worth fighting for. — **David**

Printed in Dunstable, United Kingdom